KATE SPEIR

Top 10 Crystals

Beginning your Collection and Incorporating Crystals into your Daily Routine

This book was professionally typeset on Reedsy.
Find out more at reedsy.com

"Always look for the magic which makes
the ordinary extraordinary."

-Jill Wintersteen, Spirit Daughter

Contents

1

Introduction

Welcome to a journey of transformation and empowerment, where the ancient wisdom of crystals converges with the dynamic energy of modern living. In the pages that follow, we will explore the mystical allure and practical benefits of incorporating crystals into your daily life. I'm thrilled to guide you through a path that has captivated humanity for centuries and unveil the secrets that lie within the radiant world of crystals.

Imagine holding in your hands a piece of Earth's history—a crystalline masterpiece that has witnessed the ebb and flow of time. Crystals, those exquisite gems forged deep within the belly of the Earth, have woven themselves into the tapestry of human civilization. From the opulent chambers of ancient pharaohs to the serene temples of the Far East, crystals have adorned the realms of kings and mystics alike. Their historical significance is nothing short of magical, symbolizing purity, power, and profound connection to the cosmic forces that govern our existence.

Now, let's delve into the energetic dance of crystals—the subtle frequencies that resonate with the very essence of our being. Just as a finely tuned instrument produces harmonious melodies, crystals vibrate with unique energies that can influence our thoughts, emotions, and overall well-being. We'll unlock the secrets behind the metaphysical properties of crystals, exploring how they can be harnessed to amplify your intentions, clear negative energy, and elevate your spiritual journey.

Picture a life where every facet is infused with the vibrancy of crystal energy. As we navigate the hustle and bustle of the modern world, the incorporation of crystals into our daily routines becomes a beacon of serenity and balance. From enhancing focus and creativity to fostering emotional resilience, the benefits are boundless. Together, we will uncover practical strategies for seamlessly integrating crystals into your day, empowering you to harness their potent energies and manifest positive change in your life.

In this book, I will quickly introduce you to the everyday powers for Crystals. Use this guide to help you begin your learning process. Listen to the vibrations in your body and jump to the chapter that is helpful for you in that moment. Are you feeling overwhelmed by your day and a little off, lean into the protective stone "Black Tourmaline" chapter. Needing some extra encouragement to start your day, try the motivator stone "Carnelian" chapter to get your mind ready for the day. Just looking to expand your knowledge? Then take your time and soak it all in, page by page.

Get ready to embark on a transformative expedition where the ancient whispers of crystals converge with the dynamic rhythm of your modern existence. Let the journey begin!

2

Getting Started with Crystals

Understanding Crystal Energy

Picture this: you are an energy being, and so are crystals. When you bring the two together, it's like a dance of frequencies. Crystals can absorb, store, and emit energy. Understanding how they interact with your unique energy field is the first step to unlocking their potential.

Crystals aren't a one-size-fits-all solution. Just like your goals and dreams, each crystal carries its own vibration and purpose. Whether you're seeking clarity, abundance, or love, choosing crystals aligned with your personal intentions is key to manifesting your desires.

Choosing Your First Crystals

With crystals, success shouldn't break the bank. There are plenty of budget-friendly crystal options that pack a punch. From amethyst to clear quartz, these gems won't just empower your journey; they'll do it without burning a hole in your wallet.

Ever wonder why some crystals come in different shapes and colors? Each variation carries its own unique energy signature. Whether it's a pointed crystal for focus or a soothing blue hue for calmness, understanding shapes and colors will elevate your crystal game.

Caring for Your Crystals

Just like your body needs a shower, crystals need a cleanse. Learn the art of purifying their energy and recharging them for optimal performance. Trust me; your crystals will thank you.

Is there a full moon coming up? Set your crystals outside or in your window seal and let them recharge with the power of the moon. My personal favorite is to take my crystals with me on a hike and cleanse them in the flowing rivers in Colorado. Natural water sources help connect you to the earth. Another technique which works for both your crystals and your home is to cleanse them by burning sage, open all your windows, invite the fresh air in as you waft the smoke of the burning sage over your crystals encouraging all negative energies to leave through that open window.

Your crystals are like precious gems, and proper storage is crucial to maintain their energy. Avoid exposing them to direct sunlight for extended periods, as it may fade their vibrant colors. Consider storing them in a cool, dark place, like a wooden box or a pouch, to protect them from external energies.

Having an altar near your bed or in your room will allow you to display your beautiful crystals, especially the specific ones you are calling to each day. This altar could also incorporate affirmation cards, candles, plants, and oils.

When handling your crystals, treat them with care. Remember, these beauties have been forming over millions of years. Cleanse your hands before touching them, and if you've had a particularly intense day, consider cleansing your own energy before interacting with your crystals.

So now that you've completed the first steps in your crystal journey. Get ready to unlock a new level of energy and success. Remember, the universe is abundant, and so are you. Embrace the power of crystals, and let's create the life you deserve!

3

Clear Quartz - The Master Healer

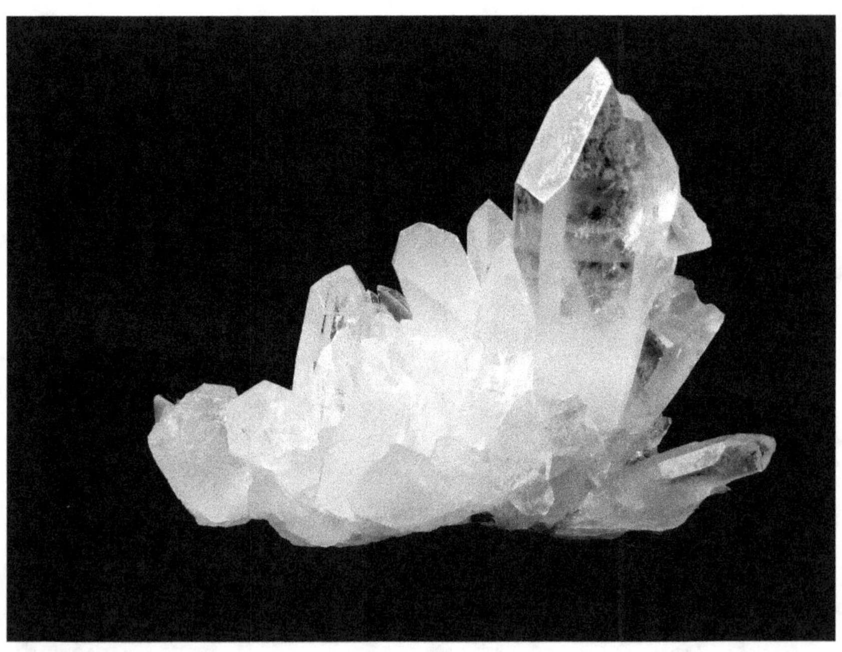

Many believe a positive mindset often emphasizes the power of clarity in achieving success and well-being. In this chapter, we delve into the world of Clear Quartz, the

Master Healer, exploring its remarkable properties and practical uses that can bring clarity and amplify positive intentions into our daily lives.

Overview of Clear Quartz Properties

Clear Quartz, with its crystal-clear appearance, is not just a visually stunning gemstone; it is a powerhouse of energy and healing. Known as the Master Healer, Clear Quartz is revered for its ability to amplify and purify energy. It is a silicon dioxide mineral that forms in a variety of crystal structures, each contributing to its unique properties.

One of the standout features of Clear Quartz is its ability to absorb, store, and release energy. This makes it an excellent tool for enhancing mental clarity, spiritual growth, and emotional balance. Whether you are a seasoned crystal enthusiast or a newcomer to the world of gemstones, Clear Quartz is a must-have in any collection.

Practical Uses for Clear Quartz in Daily Life

Meditation and Focus: In the fast-paced world we live in, finding moments of stillness and focus can be a challenge. Clear Quartz, however, acts as a beacon of tranquility. When used during meditation, it helps to clear the mind of clutter and distractions, allowing you to delve into a deeper state of awareness.

The importance of mastering your mind to achieve success is often talked about. Clear Quartz can be your ally in this journey, assisting you in gaining mental clarity and sharpening your focus. Hold a Clear Quartz crystal in your hand during meditation, and let its energy guide you towards a serene and centered state of mind.

Amplifying Intentions: People frequently emphasize the power of setting clear intentions to manifest desired outcomes. Clear Quartz serves as an amplifier for these intentions, magnifying the energy you put into your goals. Whether you're working towards personal development, career success, or improved relationships, Clear Quartz can enhance the positive energy you invest in these endeavors.

To harness the amplifying power of Clear Quartz, create an intention-setting ritual. Hold the crystal in your hand, close your eyes, and visualize your goals with utmost clarity. As you infuse the crystal with your intentions, feel the energy radiating from the quartz magnifying and empowering your desires. Keep the charged crystal in a prominent place as a daily reminder of your aspirations.

When working on your personal growth, there is a significance of consistent habits. Incorporating Clear Quartz into your daily routine, especially during moments of reflection and goal-setting, can become a powerful habit that propels you towards success.

A bonus attribute, Clear Quartz is a great crystal when using crystal combinations. Combining your Clear Quartz with another crystal you are working with will help amplify that crystal's powers. As you embark on your journey of personal growth, let the Master Healer guide you towards a clearer, more focused, and intentional life.

4

Amethyst - The Intuitive Stone

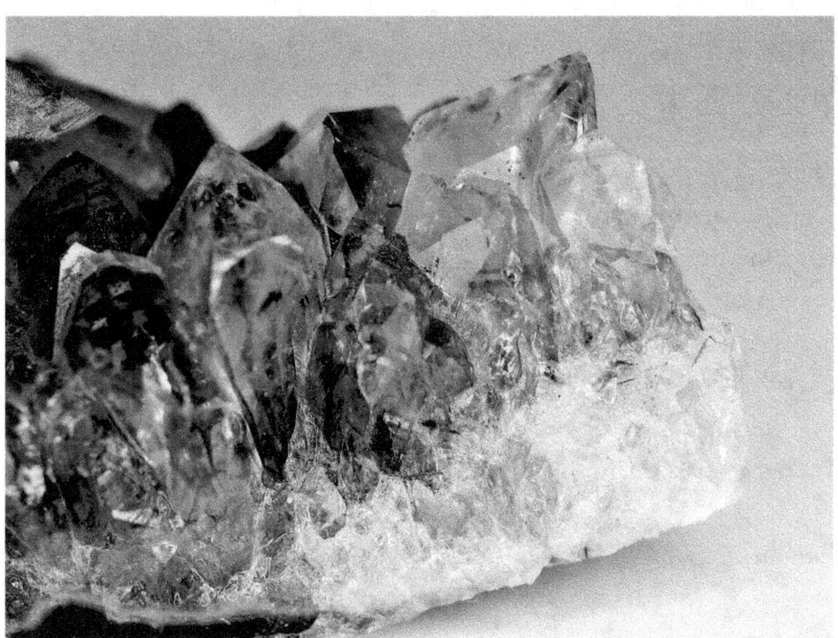

A methyst is the intuitive stone that holds the power to elevate
your life to new heights. As we unravel the secrets of this
magnificent gem, get ready to infuse your daily rituals with

the energy of Amethyst and unlock the doors to enhanced intuition, spiritual connection, restful sleep, and relaxation.

Overview of Amethyst Properties

Picture this: a vibrant purple jewel, resonating with the wisdom of the ages. Amethyst, a true powerhouse among crystals, is renowned for its ability to stimulate the mind and soothe the soul. As we embark on this journey, let's delve into the key properties that make Amethyst a game-changer in the world of spirituality.

Amethyst is a crystal of spiritual growth and protection. Its calming energy assists in overcoming stress and promoting a sense of balance. This gem acts as a conduit between the physical and spiritual realms, encouraging a harmonious integration of mind, body, and spirit.

The radiant purple hue of Amethyst is no accident; it symbolizes royalty, wisdom, and enlightenment. This regal crystal has been cherished for centuries by spiritual seekers and leaders alike. Its presence is believed to purify the aura, providing a protective shield against negative energies.

Incorporating Amethyst into Daily Rituals

Enhancing Intuition and Spiritual Connection: Imagine having a secret weapon in your arsenal that sharpens your intuition and deepens your spiritual connection. Amethyst, dear readers, is that very weapon. It is said, the power of intuition is a force that can guide you towards success and fulfillment.

Begin your day by placing Amethyst near your meditation space. Allow its energy to open the channels of intuition, heightening your awareness and decision-making abilities. As you meditate, envision the vibrant purple light surrounding you, creating a cocoon of spiritual protection and insight.

Carry a small Amethyst crystal in your pocket or wear it as jewelry throughout the day. Let its energy serve as a constant reminder to trust your instincts and tap into your inner wisdom. Whether you're navigating professional decisions or personal relationships, Amethyst is your ally in making intuitive choices that lead to greatness.

Improving Sleep and Relaxation: In the pursuit of success, it's essential to recharge your batteries. Sleep is not just a necessity; it's a pillar of peak performance. Amethyst, with its tranquil energy, becomes your sleep companion, transforming your nightly routine into a rejuvenating experience.

Create a bedtime ritual by placing Amethyst under your pillow or on your bedside table. As you unwind from the day, let the soothing energy of this crystal wash away tension and stress. Allow its gentle vibrations to lull you into a deep and restful sleep, preparing you for the challenges and triumphs that await in the morning.

As you continue in your crystal journey, you may find the importance of creating rituals to help shape your life. Incorporate Amethyst into your evening routine, and watch as your sleep improves, paving the way for greater focus, energy, and resilience during your waking hours.

Amethyst, the intuitive stone, is a valuable ally on your journey to personal mastery. Harness its properties to sharpen your intuition, deepen your spiritual connection, and cultivate restful sleep. As you infuse your daily rituals with the energy of Amethyst, remember: you are not just building routines; you are sculpting the masterpiece of your life. Embrace the power of Amethyst and elevate your existence to extraordinary heights.

5

Rose Quartz - The Stone of Love

In this chapter, we're diving into the heartwarming embrace of Rose Quartz, the Stone of Love. Get ready to explore the enchanting properties of this gentle yet powerful crystal and learn how to infuse your life with love, starting from within.

Overview of Rose Quartz Properties

Picture a soft pink gem that radiates warmth and tenderness—that's Rose Quartz. This magnificent crystal is not just a symbol of romantic love; it's a beacon of unconditional love, compassion, and harmony. As we embark on this journey, let's unravel the key properties that make Rose Quartz a transformative force in the realm of personal development.

Rose Quartz is the ultimate heart healer. Its gentle energy penetrates deep into the heart chakra, dissolving emotional wounds and inviting a sense of tranquility. This crystal resonates with the frequency of love, fostering self-love, compassion, and empathy. Rose Quartz empowers you to embrace and heal the emotional landscape within.

Using Rose Quartz for Self-Love and Relationships

Creating a Love-Infused Environment: Imagine living in an environment that exudes love and harmony. Rose Quartz, with its loving vibrations, allows you to manifest just that. Place Rose Quartz crystals strategically in your home—on your bedside table, in the living room, or on your workspace. Let these crystals serve as reminders to infuse every moment with love.

Remember, your environment shapes your destiny. Surround yourself with the loving energy of Rose Quartz to create a space that nurtures positive relationships and fosters a deep sense of connection. Whether you're single or in a relationship, let the ambiance of love created by Rose Quartz be a constant source of inspiration and joy.

Enhancing Self-Care Practices: Self-love is the foundation of a fulfilling life. Rose Quartz, the champion of self-love, guides you on a journey inward. Incorporate this gentle crystal into your self-care practices to amplify the love you give yourself. During meditation, hold Rose Quartz close to your heart and visualize the pink light enveloping you in a cocoon of unconditional love.

We all know the importance of taking care of your physical and emotional well-being, let Rose Quartz be your partner in self-care. Create a self-love ritual by placing Rose Quartz in your bath, infusing the water with its loving energy. Allow the crystal to remind you that you are worthy of love and deserve to be treated with kindness and compassion.

Rose Quartz, the Stone of Love, is a transformative ally on your journey to cultivating love within and around you. Embrace its loving energy to heal emotional wounds, create a love-infused environment, and enhance your self-care practices. As you incorporate Rose Quartz into your daily life, remember: love is not just an emotion; it's a powerful force that propels you toward a life of joy, fulfillment, and authentic connections. Let the love of Rose Quartz be the guiding light on your path to a heart-centered existence.

6

Citrine - The Abundance Stone

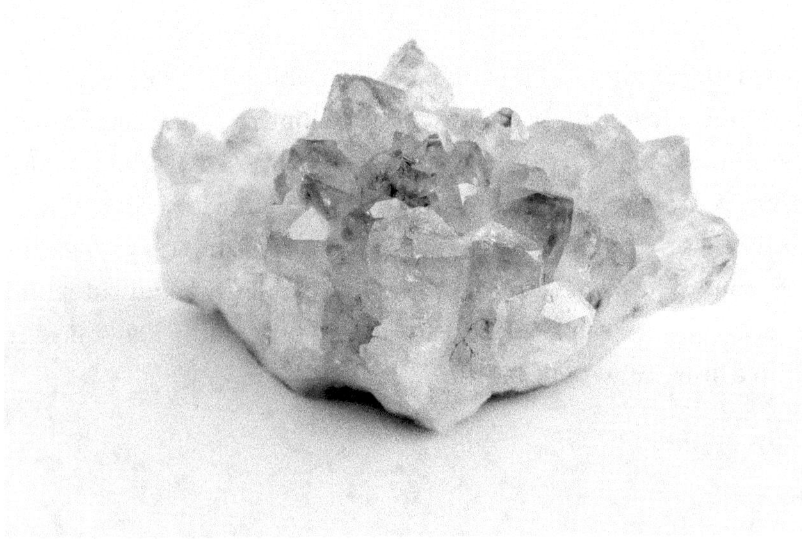

In this chapter, we embark on a journey into the golden glow of Citrine, the Abundance Stone. Prepare to discover the transformative properties of this radiant crystal and learn how to harness its power to attract prosperity and success into your life.

Overview of Citrine Properties

Imagine holding in your hands a golden gem that embodies the essence of abundance. That's Citrine—an electrifying crystal that radiates positivity and wealth. As we delve into the world of Citrine, let's explore the key properties that make it the go-to stone for those seeking abundance and prosperity.

Citrine is often referred to as the merchant's stone or the success stone. Its sunny disposition clears away negative energies, paving the way for a flow of abundance and positive vibrations. This crystal is a powerful ally in overcoming financial challenges, promoting success in business ventures, and attracting prosperity on all levels.

Believe it or not, your mindset shapes your reality. Citrine, with its uplifting energy, aligns your mindset with abundance, opening the floodgates to opportunities and success. Let's explore how you can leverage the power of Citrine to manifest your dreams.

Attracting Abundance and Prosperity with Citrine

Manifestation Techniques: There is a strong importance of clarity in goal setting and manifestation. Citrine, the ultimate abundance stone, amplifies your intentions and accelerates the manifestation process. Begin by holding a Citrine crystal in your hands during meditation or visualization exercises. As you close your eyes, focus on your goals, and let the golden energy of Citrine infuse your visions with abundance.

Create a Citrine manifestation grid by placing several Citrine crystals in a geometric pattern. As you gaze at the grid, visualize your goals as if they've already been achieved. Let the energy of Citrine magnify your intentions, sending a powerful message to the universe that you are ready to receive abundance.

Wealth and Success Rituals: Citrine is not just a passive observer; it's an active partner in your pursuit of wealth and success. Incorporate Citrine into daily rituals that align with your financial goals. Remember when we discussed the power of routines earlier in this book, infuse your morning routine with Citrine energy by holding the crystal while setting positive affirmations for a prosperous day.

Create a wealth altar by placing Citrine crystals alongside symbols of your financial goals, such as a vision board or representations of success. Regularly charge the space with the vibrant energy of Citrine, reinforcing your commitment to attracting abundance.

Citrine, the Abundance Stone, is your golden ticket to a life of prosperity and success. Embrace its energy to manifest your dreams, adopt abundance-focused mindset shifts, and infuse your daily rituals with the vibrancy of Citrine. As you embark on this journey, remember: abundance is not just about financial wealth; it's a holistic state of thriving in all aspects of your life. Let Citrine be your guiding light as you step into a world of limitless possibilities and unparalleled success.

7

Black Tourmaline - The Protective Shield

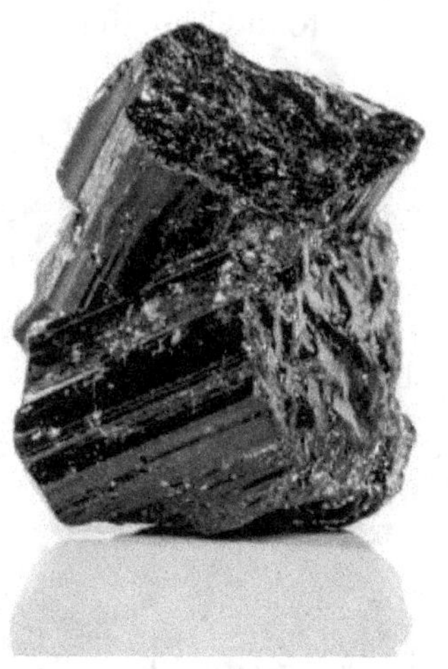

I n this chapter we're delving into the sturdy embrace of Black Tourmaline, the Protective Shield that stands guard against negative energies. Brace yourselves to uncover the powerful properties of this formidable crystal and learn how to fortify your life against unwanted influences.

Overview of Black Tourmaline Properties

Imagine holding in your hands a jet-black guardian that shields you from the storms of negativity. That's Black Tourmaline—a powerhouse of protective energy. As we navigate through the realm of this formidable crystal, let's unravel the key properties that make Black Tourmaline the go-to stone for creating a protective shield.

Black Tourmaline is a grounding stone with the ability to absorb and repel negative energies. Its dark, opaque exterior acts as a shield, deflecting unwanted vibrations and safeguarding your energetic well-being. This crystal is not just a defender; it's a warrior that anchors you to the earth, providing a solid foundation in the face of life's challenges.

Success requires not just internal strength but the ability to navigate external influences. Black Tourmaline, with its protective properties, becomes your steadfast ally in maintaining a resilient and focused mindset. Let's explore how you can harness the energy of Black Tourmaline to shield yourself from negativity.

Shielding Yourself from Negative Energies

Grounding and Protection Exercises: In the pursuit of greatness, it's crucial to stand firm in the face of adversity. Black Tourmaline, the guardian of grounded energy, assists you in maintaining your footing amidst the chaos. Incorporate grounding exercises into your daily routine by holding Black Tourmaline in your hands during meditation.

Do you believe in the power of physical anchors to shift your state?

Carry a small Black Tourmaline in your pocket as a grounding talisman. Whenever you feel overwhelmed or encounter negativity, hold the crystal and take a few deep breaths, allowing the stabilizing energy of Black Tourmaline to restore your balance.

Creating a Protective Energy Grid: While learning to create a supportive environment, Black Tourmaline empowers you to build a protective energy grid around you. Place Black Tourmaline crystals at the four corners of your living space to create a protective shield that prevents negative energies from infiltrating your sanctuary.

Enhance your workspace with Black Tourmaline to shield yourself from the stress and pressures of the outside world. As you set goals and work towards success, let the protective energy of Black Tourmaline be the fortress that preserves your focus and shields you from distractions.

Black Tourmaline, the Protective Shield, is your loyal defender in the journey of life. Embrace its grounding energy to stand resilient against negative influences, and let its protective shield become the armor that keeps you focused on your path to success. As you integrate Black Tourmaline into your life, remember: protection is not a sign of weakness but a testament to your commitment to thrive amidst any challenge. Let Black Tourmaline be the unwavering shield that propels you towards uncharted heights of success and fulfillment.

8

Selenite - The Purifier

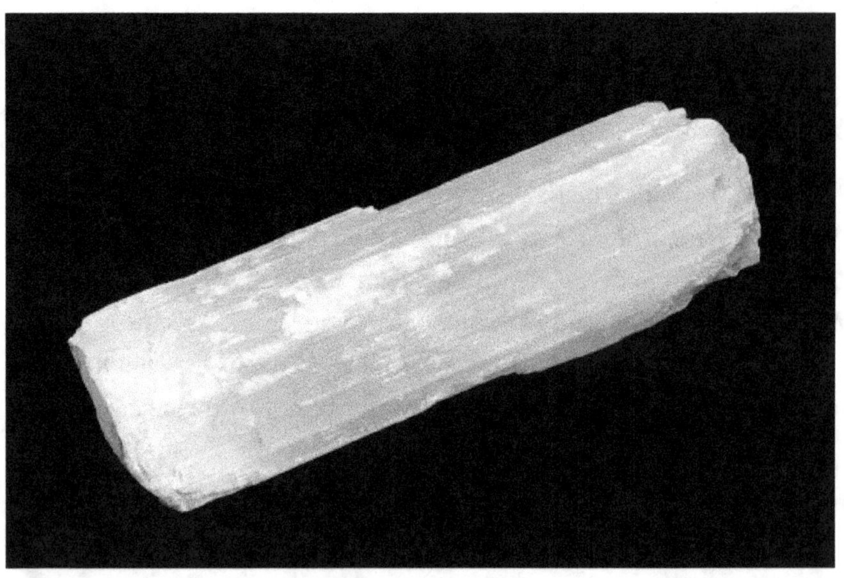

I n this chapter we embark on a transformative journey into the radiant realm of Selenite, the Purifier. Picture a crystal that serves as a beacon of purity, cleansing your energetic field and illuminating the path to clarity and spiritual awakening. Get ready to explore the captivating properties of Selenite and learn how to purify your surroundings, enhance your energy, and amplify the power of other crystals.

Overview of Selenite Properties

Imagine holding in your hands a crystal so pure and luminous that it seems to capture the essence of divine light. That's Selenite—a gem revered for its ethereal properties. As we delve into the enchanting world of Selenite, let's unravel the key characteristics that make it the go-to crystal for purification and spiritual enlightenment.

Selenite is a high-vibrational crystal that resonates with the frequencies of the higher realms. Its name is derived from Selene, the Greek goddess of the moon, emphasizing its connection to divine illumination. Selenite possesses the unique ability to cleanse and purify energy fields, making it an invaluable tool for those seeking spiritual clarity and a fresh start.

In navigating life, remember the importance of clarity and focus, Selenite becomes your ally in cutting through the noise and elevating your consciousness. Let's explore how you can harness the purifying energy of Selenite to create a space of clarity and amplify your spiritual journey.

Cleansing and Purifying Your Energy Field

Clearing Spaces and Environments: In the pursuit of success and fulfillment, it's vital to operate from a space of clarity and purity. Selenite, with its purifying energy, becomes your secret weapon in creating environments that foster focus and positive energy. Place Selenite wands strategically in your home or office to cleanse and purify the energy of the space.

As we previously discussed the impact of your environment on mindset, use Selenite to clear any stagnant or negative energy from your surroundings. Take a Selenite wand and trace the outline of your body, envisioning the crystal's radiant light purifying your energy field. Allow the calming energy of Selenite to create a sacred space for inspiration and clarity.

Amplifying the Energy of Other Crystals: Just as we mentioned the bonus quality Clear Quartz can have with collaboration, Selenite is also a team player in the crystal kingdom. Use Selenite to amplify the energy of other crystals by placing them on a Selenite charging plate or grid. This purifying crystal cleanses and recharges neighboring crystals, enhancing their effectiveness and ensuring they operate at their highest potential.

Whether you're working with Amethyst for intuition or Citrine for abundance, let Selenite be the guiding light that magnifies their energies. As you create crystal grids for manifestation or meditation, incorporate Selenite to elevate the vibrational frequency of the entire array.

Selenite, the Purifier, is your key to unlocking spiritual clarity and cleansing your energetic field. Embrace its luminous energy to create pure and sacred spaces, purify your energy field, and amplify the power of other crystals. As you integrate Selenite into your spiritual journey, remember: purification is not just a process; it's a pathway to enlightenment and a life of unparalleled clarity and purpose. Let Selenite be the beacon that guides you towards the brilliance of your truest self.

9

Labradorite - The Stone of Transformation

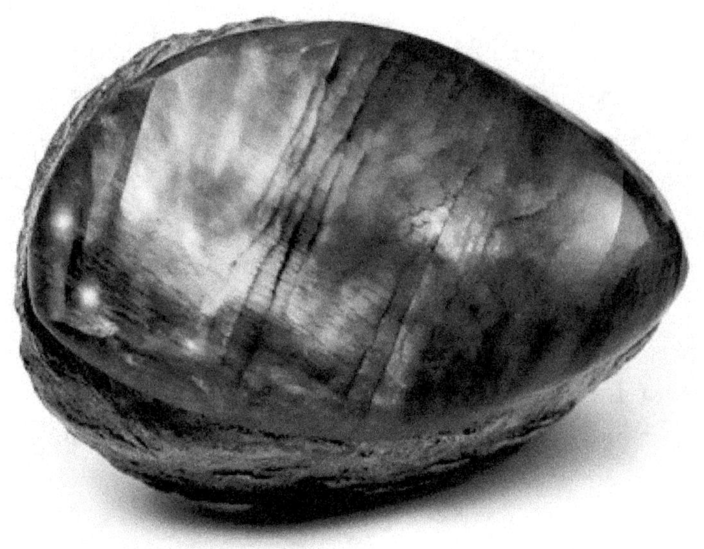

In this chapter we will explore the mesmerizing world of Labradorite, the Stone of Transformation. Imagine holding in your hands a gem that shimmers with the mysteries of the cosmos—a crystal that ignites the flames of change and propels you towards your highest potential. Get ready to explore the enchanting properties of Labradorite and learn how to embrace change, achieve your goals, and unlock a wealth of creativity and intuition within.

Overview of Labradorite Properties

Picture a stone that captures the essence of the Northern Lights, shimmering with hues of blue, green, and gold—that's Labradorite. This mesmerizing crystal is not just a feast for the eyes; it's a catalyst for profound transformation. As we delve into the world of Labradorite, let's uncover the key properties that make it the ultimate stone for personal growth and evolution.

Labradorite is a stone of magic and mystery, resonating with the energies of transformation and self-discovery. Its iridescent sheen reflects the ever-changing nature of life, reminding us to embrace change as a catalyst for growth. Labradorite is a powerful ally in navigating life's transitions, helping us release old patterns and step into the unknown with courage and confidence.

Change is not something to be feared but embraced as an opportunity for growth. Labradorite becomes your guide in the journey of transformation, empowering you to tap into your inner strength and unleash your full potential.

Embracing Change and Personal Growth with Labradorite

Setting and Achieving Goals: In the pursuit of success, it's essential to set bold goals and take inspired action. Labradorite, with its transformative energy, becomes your ally in manifesting your dreams. Begin by holding Labradorite in your hands during goal-setting sessions, allowing its vibrant energy to infuse your intentions with clarity and purpose.

Use Labradorite to refine your objectives and create a clear path. Let its mystical energy ignite the fire of motivation within you, propelling you towards your goals with unwavering determination.

Enhancing Creativity and Intuition: Creativity and intuition are the cornerstones of innovation and success. Labradorite, the stone of transformation, amplifies these innate qualities, unlocking the door to unlimited creative potential and intuitive insights. Incorporate Labradorite into your creative endeavors by placing it on your workspace or wearing it as jewelry.

We are often greeted with the power of intuition in decision-making, let Labradorite be your intuitive guide. During meditation or quiet reflection, hold Labradorite close to your heart and invite its mystical energy to awaken your inner wisdom. Trust in the guidance that emerges, knowing that Labradorite is guiding you towards transformative breakthroughs.

Labradorite, the Stone of Transformation, is your partner in the journey of personal growth and evolution. Embrace its mystical energy to navigate life's changes with courage and confidence, set and achieve bold goals, and unlock your creative potential and intuitive insights. As you integrate Labradorite into your life, remember: transformation is not just a destination but a journey of self-discovery and empowerment. Let Labradorite be the guiding light that leads you towards a life of limitless possibilities and profound fulfillment.

<h1 style="text-align:center">10</h1>

Carnelian - The Motivator

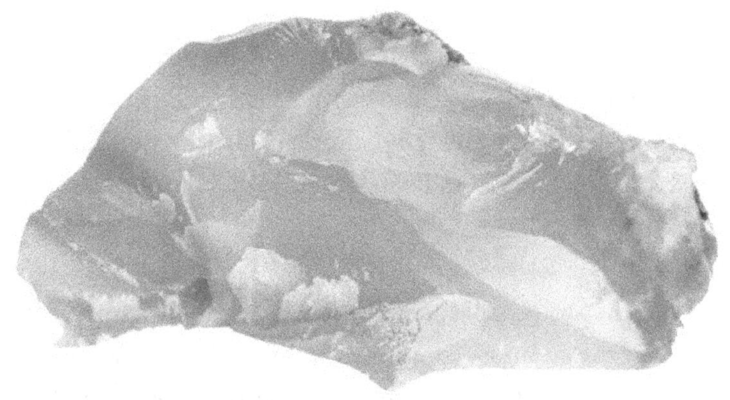

Carnelian, the Motivator—a gem that pulses with the fiery energy of motivation and vitality. Imagine holding in your hands a crystal that ignites the flames of ambition and propels you towards peak performance. Get ready to explore the invigorating properties of Carnelian and learn how to infuse your daily routine with motivation, boost your vitality, and harness its dynamic energy for enhanced productivity and creativity.

Overview of Carnelian Properties

Visualize a gem that embodies the warmth of a sunset, radiating with shades of orange and red—that's Carnelian. This dynamic crystal is not just a feast for the eyes; it's a catalyst for motivation and vitality. As we delve into the world of Carnelian, let's uncover the key properties that make it the ultimate stone for boosting energy, motivation, and drive.

Carnelian is a stone of action and ambition, resonating with the energies of passion and determination. Its vibrant hues mirror the fiery spirit it imparts to those who embrace its energy. Carnelian is known for its ability to stimulate creativity, enhance motivation, and fuel a zest for life. As the power of energy and passion leads to achieving success, Carnelian becomes your ally in unlocking your full potential.

Boosting Motivation and Vitality

Incorporating Carnelian into Your Daily Routine: In the pursuit of a fulfilling life, a daily routine that fosters motivation is key. Carnelian, the Motivator, seamlessly integrates into your rituals, infusing each moment with a burst of energy. Begin your day by wearing Carnelian jewelry or carrying a small Carnelian stone in your pocket. Allow its dynamic energy to awaken your senses and set the tone for a day filled with motivation and vitality.

Remember the importance of morning routines, make Carnelian a centerpiece of your waking ritual. Hold the crystal in your hands and visualize your goals with vivid clarity. Let the energy of Carnelian propel you into the day with a sense of purpose and determination.

Harnessing its Energy for Productivity and Creativity: Productivity and creativity are the building blocks of success. Carnelian, with its invigorating energy, becomes the catalyst for unlocking your creative potential and boosting productivity. Place Carnelian on your workspace or carry it with you during brainstorming sessions to enhance your creative thinking.

In life, there is a power in your state of mind management. Use Carnelian to shift your state when faced with challenges or moments of fatigue. Hold the crystal in your hands, close your eyes, and let its vibrant energy revitalize your spirit. As you re-engage with tasks, feel the surge of motivation and vitality propelling you towards peak performance.

Carnelian, the Motivator, is your secret weapon in the pursuit of peak performance and success. Embrace its dynamic energy to infuse motivation and vitality into your daily routine, and let its fiery spirit propel you towards your goals. As you integrate Carnelian into your life, remember: motivation is not just a fleeting emotion; it's a dynamic force that propels you towards your aspirations. Let Carnelian be the driving force that transforms your ambitions into achievements and fuels your journey towards unparalleled success.

Hematite - The Grounding Stone

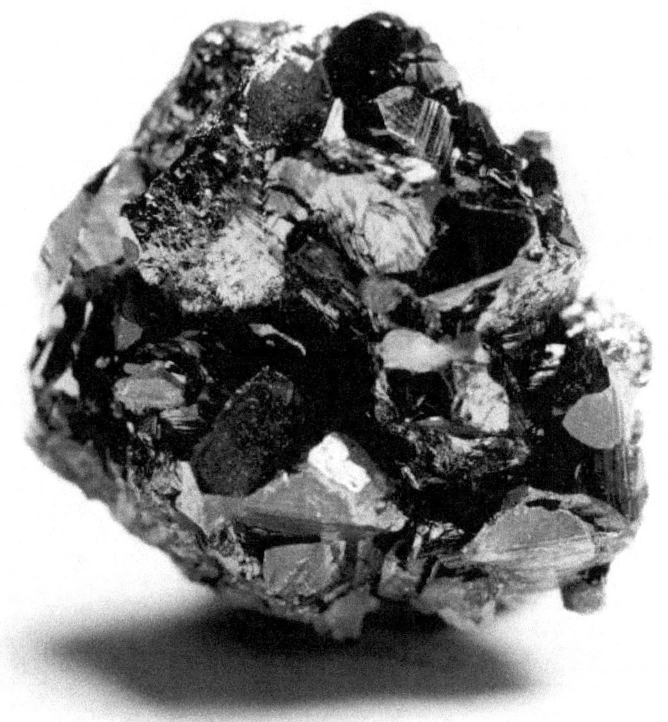

Here, we will look at the unyielding embrace of Hematite, the Grounding Stone—a gem that anchors you to the earth, stabilizing your energy and fostering a sense of balance. Picture a metallic sheen reflecting the strength within; that's Hematite, a formidable ally in grounding emotions, reducing stress, and enhancing mental clarity. Get ready to explore the grounding properties of Hematite and learn how to cultivate emotional resilience, mental focus, and an unshakable foundation for success.

Overview of Hematite Properties

Imagine holding a stone that mirrors the strength and resilience of solid iron—that's Hematite. This metallic-gray crystal is not just visually striking; it's a powerhouse of grounding energy. As we venture into the world of Hematite, let's unravel the key properties that make it the ultimate stone for grounding and stabilizing your energy.

Hematite is a grounding force that aligns your energy with the frequency of the Earth. Its reflective surface symbolizes the clarity and focus it brings to those who embrace its energy. Hematite is renowned for its ability to absorb negative energy, providing a protective shield that fosters emotional balance and mental stability.

When remembering the importance of emotional resilience and mental focus, Hematite becomes your steadfast companion in navigating the challenges of life. Let's explore how you can harness the grounding energy of Hematite to cultivate emotional stability and enhance mental clarity.

Grounding and Stabilizing Your Energy

Balancing Emotions and Reducing Stress: In the pursuit of success, emotional balance is a crucial foundation. Hematite, the Grounding Stone, assists you in cultivating emotional resilience and reducing stress. Incorporate Hematite into your daily routine by wearing it as jewelry or carrying a small Hematite stone in your pocket.

When you emphasize the importance of managing emotions, use Hematite to create a grounding ritual during moments of stress. Hold the crystal in your hands and visualize the calming energy of Hematite flowing through you, grounding and stabilizing your emotions. Allow its protective shield to absorb any negativity, leaving you with a sense of inner peace.

Enhancing Mental Clarity and Focus: Mental clarity is the cornerstone of effective decision-making and focus. Hematite, with its stabilizing energy, becomes your ally in enhancing mental clarity and sharpening focus. Place Hematite on your desk or carry it with you during work or study sessions to create a grounded and focused mindset.

As mentioned earlier, crystals can help harness your power of state management. Use Hematite to shift your mental state from chaos to clarity. Hold the crystal in your hands, close your eyes, and allow its grounding energy to anchor your thoughts. Feel the mental fog lifting, leaving you with enhanced focus and the ability to tackle tasks with precision.

Hematite, the Grounding Stone, is your rock-solid foundation for emotional stability and mental clarity. Embrace its grounding energy to balance your emotions, reduce stress, and enhance focus. As you integrate Hematite into your life, remember: stability is not a sign of weakness but a testament to your resilience and strength. Let Hematite be the unyielding anchor that grounds you amidst the storms, allowing you to rise to new heights with unwavering stability and focus.

12

Amazonite - The Stone of Serenity & Luck

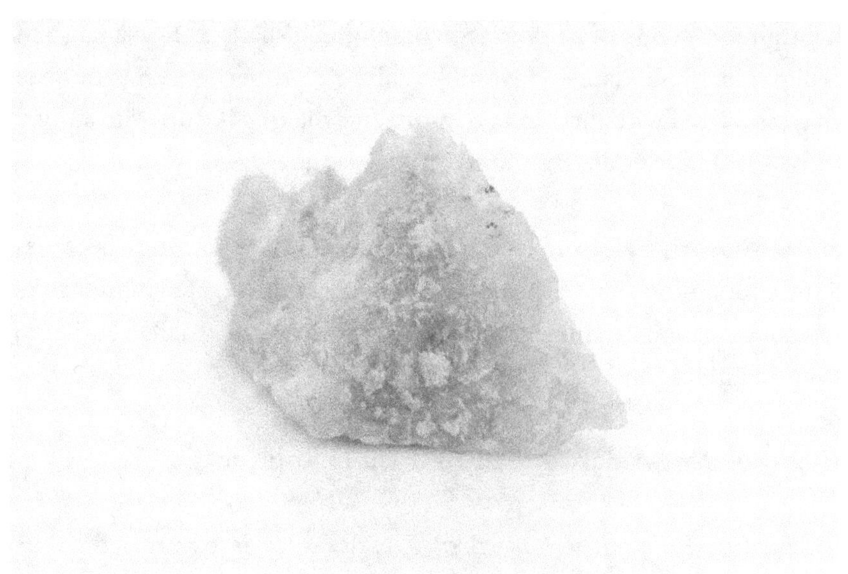

In this chapter, we're delving into the enchanting world of Amazonite, often referred to as the Gambler's Stone. Imagine holding in your hands a gem that echoes the spirit of fortune, a crystal that invites luck and soothes the soul. Get ready to explore the properties of Amazonite and discover how to infuse your daily routine with its soothing and luck-attracting energies.

Overview of Amazonite Properties

Picture a stone that mirrors the lush green hues of the Amazon rainforest—that's Amazonite. This captivating crystal is not just a visual delight; it's a talisman of luck and serenity. As we venture into the world of Amazonite, let's unravel the key properties that make it the ultimate stone for those who thrive on taking risks and embracing uncertainty.

Amazonite is known for its soothing and calming energy, resembling the tranquil waters of a River. Its vibrant green shade exudes a sense of renewal and abundance. Beyond its calming properties, Amazonite is also associated with luck and good fortune, making it a favorite among those seeking a bit of serendipity in their endeavors.

Seizing opportunities and embracing uncertainty? Amazonite becomes your companion in navigating the unpredictable journey of life. Let's explore how you can incorporate Amazonite into your daily routine to invite calmness and good luck into your life.

Incorporating Amazonite in Your Daily Routine

Soothing and Calming Properties: Life is a series of unpredictable events, and maintaining a sense of calm amidst chaos is essential. Amazonite, with its soothing energy, becomes your anchor in the storm. Incorporate Amazonite into your daily routine by wearing it as jewelry, placing it on your desk, or carrying a small Amazonite stone in your pocket.

While maintaining a peak state, use Amazonite to create a calming ritual during moments of stress or uncertainty. Hold the crystal in your hands, close your eyes, and visualize the gentle, flowing energy of a river washing away tension and leaving you in a state of serene calmness.

Good Luck or Fortune: Life is a gamble, and sometimes a bit of luck can make all the difference. Amazonite, known as the Gambler's Stone, is believed to attract good luck and fortune. Integrate Amazonite into your daily routine to infuse your endeavors with positive energy and serendipity.

Tune into the power of positive thinking, use Amazonite as a touchstone for optimism and luck. Carry it with you during important life events or decision-making moments. Allow its energy to be a reminder that, like the river that flows steadily, luck and fortune can find their way into your life.

Amazonite, the Stone of Serenity and Luck, is your lucky charm in the game of life. Embrace its soothing and luck-attracting energy to navigate uncertainty with calmness and invite positive outcomes into your endeavors. As you integrate Amazonite into your daily routine, remember: luck is not just a chance event; it's a state of being that you can cultivate. Let Amazonite be the river of fortune that flows through your life, bringing serenity and luck to every twist and turn.

13

Conclusion

We have embarked on a journey through the dazzling world of crystals, each gem a beacon of energy and potential. As we close the book, let's recap the wisdom of the top 10 crystals that can transform your life.

1. Clear Quartz - The Amplifier: Harness its clarity to magnify your intentions and amplify your energy.
2. Amethyst - The Intuitive Stone: Elevate your life with enhanced intuition, spiritual connection, and restful sleep.
3. Rose Quartz - The Stone of Love: Cultivate love within and around you, creating a harmonious and joyful existence.
4. Citrine - The Abundance Stone: Attract prosperity and success into your life by manifesting your dreams with the golden energy of Citrine.
5. Black Tourmaline - The Protective Shield: Stand resilient against negativity, create protective energy grids, and cultivate a positive environment.
6. Selenite - The Purifier: Cleanse your surroundings, enhance intuition, and amplify the power of other crystals with the purifying

light of Selenite.

7. Labradorite - The Stone of Transformation: Embrace change, achieve your goals, and unlock creative potential with the mystical energy of Labradorite.

8. Carnelian - The Motivator: Infuse motivation and vitality into your daily routine, setting and achieving bold goals with the fiery energy of Carnelian.

9. Hematite - The Grounding Stone: Anchor your emotions, reduce stress, and enhance mental clarity with the stabilizing force of Hematite.

10. Amazonite - The Stone of Serenity & Luck: Invite serenity, good luck, and fortune into your life as you navigate uncertainties with the calming energy of Amazonite.

As you continue your exploration of crystals, let me remind you that your connection with these stones is deeply personal. Each crystal holds a unique frequency, just like you. Dive into the experience, feel the energies, and let them guide you on your journey.

I encourage you to cultivate a daily practice, integrating these crystals into your routines, and allowing their energies to become a seamless part of your life. In doing so, you'll witness the profound impact they can have on your mindset, energy, and overall well-being.

For those eager to delve deeper, consider adding to your crystal collection, carefully selecting gems that resonate with your goals and intentions. Whether through local crystal shops, online platforms, or attending gem shows, each addition to your collection is a step towards a more empowered and intentional life.

If you found this book helpful, I invite you to review your experiences on Amazon. What breakthroughs have you encountered? How has your mindset shifted? Share your insights and discoveries, as your journey may inspire and empower others.

Remember, the power lies within you, and these crystals are catalysts for unlocking that power. May your path be illuminated, your spirit uplifted, and your journey one of continuous growth and expansion.

Keep thriving, keep shining, and keep embracing the extraordinary possibilities that await you.

14

Resources

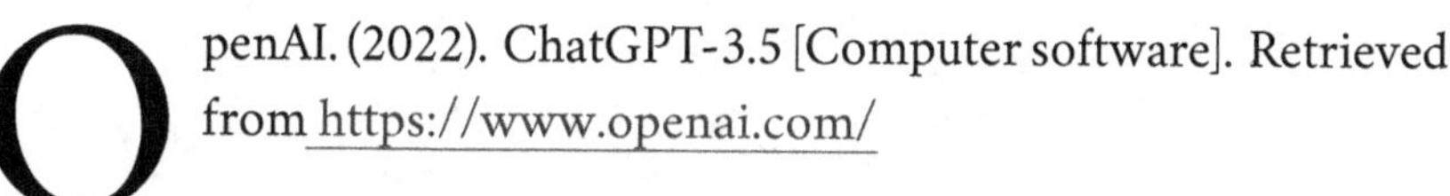OpenAI. (2022). ChatGPT-3.5 [Computer software]. Retrieved from https://www.openai.com/

www.ingramcontent.com/pod-product-compliance
Lightning Source LLC
Chambersburg PA
CBHW050750250726